I0092488

BLOODLINE

BLOODLINE

Ansley Clark

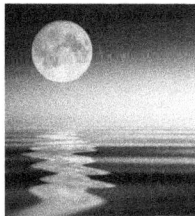

MoonPath Press

Copyright © 2024 Ansley Clark.
All rights reserved.

No part of this publication may be reproduced, distributed,
or transmitted in any form or by any means whatsoever without
written permission from the publisher, except in the case of brief
excerpts for critical reviews and articles.
All inquiries should be addressed to MoonPath Press.

Poetry
ISBN 978-1-936657-87-2

Cover art: Hannah Brancato, *Soma*, 2024:
natural dye, citric acid, embroidery thread, cotton.
www.hannahbrancato.com

Author photo: Rose Shepherd

Book design: Tonya Namura, using
Garamond Premier Pro (text) and Sofia Pro (display).

MoonPath Press, an imprint of Concrete Wolf Poetry Series, is
dedicated to publishing the finest poets living in
the U.S. Pacific Northwest.

MoonPath Press
c/o Concrete Wolf
PO Box 2220
Newport, OR 97365-0163

MoonPathPress@gmail.com

http://MoonPathPress.com

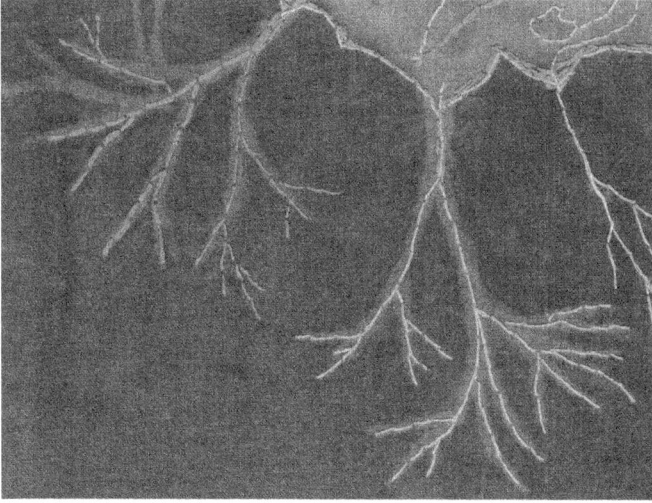

For mama

Contents

○

○

○

BLOODLINE

Sick Woman Theory maintains that the body and mind are sensitive and reactive to regimes of oppression—particularly our current regime of neoliberal, white-supremacist, imperial-capitalist, cis-hetero-patriarchy. It is that all of our bodies and minds carry the historical trauma of this...it is the world itself that is making and keeping us sick.
—Johanna Hedva

So I taught myself to be silent, I apologized for everything. I reined in my tongue, I was polite and compliant. Yet secretly I was bad. I didn't know how to calm the blood that made me potentially a fury, I was seething, and for that I tortured myself.
—Elena Ferrante

A house can be a dynasty, a bloodline, a body.
—Bettina Judd

Returning in Late Summer to the Uncanny

Salt-wet   collapsed orange   the air so full it's almost
a real live human emotion   almost clothed it   hangs

you might see a side of her that's difficult to see my father says
as a deer gallops through the fluorescent tunnel   fleeing wildfire

I've heard of deer   inside the sea's curled edge
who swim between islands   between worlds

in the weeks caring for my mother and the house
deer appear close three times   once in this fluorescent panic

then twice more standing around staring   with chilly demeanors
surely this must be a sign!   I think   opening my box

of wretched fables   but no other signs follow
leaving me to wake   with a thirst for narrative

one morning a four-poster bed arrives with the tides
heaped   with heavy blankets under which lie

a family of undetermined bodies   dead or sleeping
I am not certain   I turn away   covering my face

the real uncanny is a strange survival
finding a human presence

where it shouldn't be   like opening
the door of the house   to find another house

later my mother cries softly
in her bandages on the couch

if I must name it   this is a raw   incubatory period
a looping uneasiness stalks each pooled night

the house on its hill exposed as bristle   the wounds inside what
the stars' vacuum inhales   inhales out and up

Lineage of Power

A path through the bog
lit by an un-metaphored and green   starry feeling

climbs down   where some women keep its secret
like nettles in cloth   there is no leader here   which

confuses men   who cover their eyes and deem
certain   inclinations impossible

one woman learns mistletoe's precarious edge
and coaxes steaming cloth   another

can compel a specific animal
to pursue the male object   to ferry desire

some learn to preserve these abilities through the generations
like knives muted in wool   a line tossed in uncertain seawater

it's true that someday things will begin to die
into their hot projections

a woman will look down into a watery cathedral
and barely discern the shadows of sex

thus brambled into a mind   familiarized with restriction
this lessening will feel like the most feminine magic trick

and this fatigue a wet amulet
a battery light in an ill-lit century

where individuals purposeless   half-articulated
stand on every threshold as uncertain guests

Bloodline

There are systems in place   around us
make-believe   and real

like complicated ropes
strung through the trees

though upon looking   one always finds
a lurking disorder   like a vacant whistle

people float by dressed   in numbers and patterns
without faces   a controlled geometry

all day I have been knocking at them
I wave my bare arms   throw things

but the people keep proceeding   on their errands
to wherever   the next gathering is   whatever

the next gathering is   where bodies are free
from desire

this is all   definitely going somewhere
much like our lives

exhausted I fall quiet   in my square of dark moss
and no one comes

Americana

Every night we hear the sound
of someone running through the trees

as though something is trying to come unstuck   a trapped animal
throwing itself at the unyielding edges

when my brothers investigate they report   *no ghost here*
just the neighbor boy running back and forth in the dark

no one comments   on the strangeness
of this event   what the darkness does to a person

how the systems disconnect us   but how
little we know   about our neighbors frightens me

because some needs   are unsolvable my mother
preserves old longings in me like pressed flowers

eventually I learn it is only acceptable to have a need
if I can keep it to myself

thus when   after four days without power
I hear a phantom panting in my ear   I think

of course my ghost is wolfish hunger
and everyone knows a hunger chambered

grows deranged   desert-flung
like a voice in isolation

in the parceled land   the nation's steady vernacular
of ownership and borders   invents trespassing

at dusk a high whistle splits the tree line
unanswered   this call for an animal's return

floats   a lonely fluorescence   above our properties
now fractured   as night comes

to watch my family like all other families
participate in this system   is to feel myself panic

the future's coin spins on one edge
this has happened many times before

Container

Searching for a safe place for the mind
as something heightened   and frenetic thickens

coming apart   like an unsteady figure
on a plane of wind

a shape flees its blue   the frigid night
flares volatile   like a dangerous-feeling party

what have I wanted
some safety   a distant blue glitter

if not in love   then in
an easy controlled self

once briefly I   stopped caring
so much   it felt like   a floral dress or like   ecstatic power

I wandered home from the bar quieted and alone
boundaried   like I belonged

to myself   like something very good
might come my way   anytime   right then even

not in love with anyone   unanchored
community arose   in surprising brightness

before the rain building itself   balconied
dissolved once again the perimeter   my location slipping

Water Effect

What stays is water   fog   which by now
feels like erasure   and what is tiny anyway
certain angles of bent wrist   someone's annual
breakdown in the kitchen   the storming out of
the house   and the terror
of long silences   inside of which I arrange
myself   an empty outline
a cinnamon light   cast by lamps in skeletal circles
I fluctuate too largely   as a child   I dreamed of a man
robed   emerging   from a pool's green mist
I would call out   for a caregiver   when I could not
remember my own name   in the wet forest   sometimes
an umbrella   would burst into flame

A Childhood

A man tells me   to *go look in there*
at the carcass in the peaty undergrowth

because he knows I cannot stomach gore
says *we gotta toughen you up*   then laughs as I hide my face

so shamed I follow a white thread
like a loose nerve

while men explain violence to me
its value and nuance

in this confusing arrangement
I keep a fragment of unbecoming

looped around my wrist   I know the place
in these woods where milk drips

from an animal's eye   and systems
come apart in green fog

I am not afraid of the real you see   thus mostly
I do not think I am weak   or need to be toughened

like a kind of tempered glass
fortified to be used endlessly without shattering

it isn't the gore it is the bullet
which interrupts my education   and sexualized

into this unease   I find
a gray rag of myself   I find out

what my mouth can do with fear
then I spin   as an object does

17

A Room

Two women hold secret meetings
in the old boathouse
because there is nowhere else left
the house   so like a marriage   being full of surveillance
and when the letters disappear into
the larger governing system   can this
knowledge of a hidden space sustain?   and who is
in the interior there   looking outward
and which forest fragments will survive
shadowed and unclaimed?
a woman walks the corridors
looking for a way out
as long lines of warehouses climb
into the fog above a city   the same warehouses
creating and processing
our brimming excess   which will not
grant us freedom   nor safety
growing up   a woman lived in the woods
behind our house
now I'm trying to argue
for wasted spaces   what catches flame
what is not wanted   nor promised
to anyone   nor approved
nor required to listen

White Deer

The story goes   late one night   driving home from a party
he got lost in the woods
and turned down a long dirt road
and out of the trees   leapt two
all-white deer   *with glowing red eyes*   he said
the deer started running alongside his car
like cracks in the darkness   white flashes
swimming the night's evergreen currents
and then the deer   get this
reared up on their hind legs and turned and looked at him
I mean   they were running alongside his car on two legs
their two front legs dangling weirdly in the air
he slammed on his brakes and the deer
ran back into the woods
and that's the whole story   I'm not even sure
if I'm remembering this correctly
who saw the deer   who told the story   did anyone
tell the story?   am I
misremembering?   I remember
my brother was sick
and I had stopped eating because
I felt wary of my own joy   which seemed
obscene   and the house's silences
had lasted four days
I was sixteen   while I had
always loved the woods and the strange things
found there   I was
starting to feel afraid

The Tarp

I was a good sister   I cared for them
and I was a good daughter
in that I learned to disappear
mother figure they said   and *she's a natural*
the self being chameleonlike   starved
for category   like a floral arrangement
I coped well in a crisis
carried my brothers on my back
cradled them in my lap
with my hands over their ears
so they couldn't hear
our parents sobbing in the next room
a sound   like tissue paper tearing
and we craved   little houses
so I hung a tarp in the woods   blue shadow
blue   little house
have I been clear
enough?   I was good
for a long time   and it was a chaotic environment
and the year it rained
too much the tarp
finally yielded   and   oh how do I say this
my rage surprised me
my brother was trapped
underneath the tarp
which had collapsed under fallen branches
and he called out to me
help   an unbearable tiny voice
his lump of fragile body
struggling under the thick plastic
it was at that moment I felt a sharp tug—
like the violent urge
to throw oneself   into the deepest water
I am uncertain

as to the exact moment
when I stopped being good   this guilt
an empty shape   always moving inside me
in any case
what happened back then was
I raised my foot
above my brother beneath the tarp
and crushed the part
that looked like a face as hard as I could

Bloodline

The winter our animal dies nothing else
particularly bad happens

except I am out of my mind absorbing
the sadness around me

I think she took the cancer from my body into hers   my mother says
referring to the dog   who is currently dying by the woodstove

the whole scene and the night's   damp animal spell so
stupidly sad   I want to laugh

as always the imaginative realm approaches   kindly but
unworkably   there are many possible holes/entries

at night I lean my face
into these openings to sleep

what to do with this old family habit
of feeling shame for one's survival?   it pools at our feet

apologies for joy embroidered
in floral reds

when my brother became sick I was 16
in my body a recklessness glittered   dark as salt

I thought his illness was because I had not
been paying enough attention

the feelings they will kill me someday
the steady flow of them   into and out of my reality like thin milk

to leave would mean surrendering them to this weather
and in solitude the guilt cuts

sharp as collarbone   as hip bone
self-denial   a clear sea

asking as I have been
how long are you going to punish yourself

and where does a bloodline dry up
and where is its source

Starts to Get to Me After a While

Voices grow louder in isolation
a knotted shiver   the mind   spins
like an unsteady top
all night I hear   some clicking in the air
like lamps switching on and off
or like eyes blinking or lots of snapping legs   as a creature
weeps by the dark creek
my mother cries out at her hallucinations
and I only have one small knife
I leap from my bed
and shake my knife at nothing
a woman follows me home
a tremor arises from nothing
still   a glass house in the woods
lets too much in   I kneel and bury
my life in damp ground
on the bluff I can safely see the horizon
all that comes   then the tides carry in
many crawling black dots
and then the island on its axis
it inhales   then it wobbles

Interior vs. Exterior

Clouded signal   on fire in someone's palm
I am so   uncertain

as to whether the steady drone   is at the cellular level or is
part of the room   like an artificial light buried in the ground

what occurs inside my head is not separate
is thus hegemonically diminished

these canyons of reality built
in shining stacked blocks   the male reality

constructed and reflective
as a mirror I no longer trust

I mean even the wind
is a harsh political wind   makes me feel

like I will lose everything   as a child
I watched my mother pace and pace with work

and like the women before me I follow orders
then receive a square paper inscribed with numbers

and receive then some loneliness too
frightened into agreement

and frantic   I offer as evidence of compliance
my rectangle of insignificant

financial accounts   my tidied piece
of glowing dirt

what I see in the yard   among bottles
there was a difficult language   definitions for not belonging

Recurring Dream

I really need to have lunch with my mother
before something crawls back

a question of water
a ladder into the canyon

days descend
like small moons on a system of ropes

I don't want anyone to know
I'm in the bone flowers now   hugging the dark animal

The Hypochondriac and the Adjacent

How to explain I had a weird dream?
or that at night   something moves through the rushes
or a voice from the neighboring town   calls my name?

walking the house's perimeter I carry
receipts   miniature lists   pharmaceuticals
trace the hypothetical geometries:
if three cardinals pause on the snowy sill   if the deer appear again
I think humans devise superstitions because
they stand at an edge   controlling nothing
superstitions are like little bad prayers
attempts to control a wildness which
does or does not sense our presence
tonight an animal calls out so lonely
if it calls out again   or if it quiets

the shame of a pity object
the shame of nothing is wrong with you/the shame of
something is wrong with you
a hole in the body   where a pencil light pokes through
later the doctor's colored charts   not meant to cause fear
but to quantify or explain   invisible floating things
like a ghost inside the body
or a machine sound from the basement
meanwhile complicated equipment beeps
and someone hums   deep in the house

I acquire the habit of palpating my armpit
and my throat like soft eggs
spend most days chewing
cruciferous stalks   turmeric   black garlic
a cup of hot ginger and surely
something good will happen soon   some luminous dent
the doctor warns of letting my body waver
out of control   like an indeterminate weather
then pokes and kneads my breasts
their red lozenges   red fatty aches
the shadow spaces I am afraid to touch
deep in the lumpy tissue   perhaps a lamp
my mother buried before I was born   a warm brown rot

this self-doubt   *you will get used to it*

if we could understand our lives to have a long theme of arrival

a familiar object hovers   husk-lunged
so close I can hear it breathe
what follows follows me
underground in clear spools   unravels

Stochastic as Background Noise

A woman weeps in the hall   and I feel
like I will lose my mind

lining up suspicions   like collected stones
on the windowsill at night

moving through the murky water   pulling apart
the exposed strands as they multiply

this casual glass of wine   this bacon
which makes my mouth water

my grandmothers lived among chemicals
in a factory   my aunt above a laundromat

Sugar and meat
soy isolate protein

fat
too much fat

salt deposits in lymph nodes from
a lack of water

radioactive cell phones
anti-perspirant

alcohol   as little as
three drinks per week especially

the mind's obsessive looping   a closet
storing useless coordinates

in a recurring nightmare something
terrible is happening to a body

and the dream self doesn't want
to peel back the hands from the face to look

how many errors am I allowed to live and still
be considered good?

how long will I be   a thing to correct?
chipping away at   the parts deemed deficient

the present is a large lake   it offers
what it can and nothing else

alcohol consumed while young   a fragile period
one bad gene
several bad genes
one missing gene
rejecting motherhood
motherhood that is too late
compression for example bras
parabens
yellowed shards of longing
lack of access to health care
i.e. not being rich   or white
an unhealthy mind   negative thoughts

39

when asked if I check regularly
I lie and nod

and turn my face from myself
offer my wrists   up and out   to the dark

as in the fear of cancer

causes breast cancer   a male doctor says

so just enjoy your life   haha

a chaotic place like

a brain on fire

unmitigated restlessness

unmanageable desire

Umbilical

That force   which has become
a habit

the mired conviction in
fish bones   buried in the throat

or climbing temporary steeples   a strategy
for seeking water

which shimmers up   pale blue
from the tideflats

and I   tearing out the remaining lawn
carrying stolen meats   see her there   my mother

thin and alone at the edge of the woods
which hurts   and

keeps me here   crawling down
the tunnel of mesh light

to feed us both meat
and cold water

Ghost in the Shell Daughter

Greening copper question   *will you have children*
as the years pass   unfruitfully therefore

uneconomically   and my uncertain response
when I myself feel

no sense of self-possession here
but instead belong   to everyone who needs me

each day coming apart   beholden
to each individual or system I brush up against

I need evenings   stars calm as water
to cool and knit myself   back to a single form

trembling against   the urge to disappear
how does the self survive   when the day becomes a market

and on the long commute home
the darkness hides   the private urgencies of strangers

labor's husks sailing moonlit highways
in one apartment a woman

oils and combs her long damaged hair
believes her deep fatigue   which is the fatigue of erosion

to be instead an illusion of her tangled nerves
trash fires at her mind's periphery

I didn't realize the hardest part would be
trusting   one's own perception of reality

the hardest part   locating the ghost
when it's the 21st century   and the world

doesn't look like the world anymore
but instead like images   digital signifiers

the sky softly destabilizes
it feels like a burning

Milk

In spring a cold scrap
floats down from the sun

someone's daughter has been
squinting for hours to catch it

alone in a time
of private scarcity   harnessed

to the light wheat
of a hollow belly   a wire

knives her wrist
to the sky

truly what is   a daughter
but some loneliness

and to make of self-refusal
an energy of secrets

you seem so fragile
is what she likes to hear

this too   is a hunger
so fragile it will not listen

I Am a Bad System

Culmination of genes heavy with
recall   as one would harbor

some known light memory though it is
no longer true   I have in this life learned many varied

ways to distrust myself
from which I choose depending on the context

gray figures hover in the periphery
though I do not believe in determinism

or free will   though I believe in complication
the shadowed green of a lake

how   what's the word   claustrophobic   rectangular
to discover a structure over everything   like science fiction

beyond which is hard to imagine
like a line of white mountains in air

sometimes an outside reality bleeds through a person
and produces the same disorientation as two moons

such as   the recurring dream about a man in the dark yard trying
to get inside my house   an intensity constructs   feeds on itself

I should be a better worker but I   cry too easily   my stomach
does not look the way it should

I tell my leg to run and   aching machine it locks
I tell my face to compose itself and it reveals

a system of strong pink sadnesses   my apartment also a system
of monetary agreements   changing like clouds

I lack stamina   though worry will probably be
what gets me in the end   wouldn't that be funny

I am less real than I know   all plastic space
like a bad government   all emotion like a soft difficult thing

The Knife

In manufacturing what they call
the perfect system   they create a problem

out of ourselves   and the problem
it is infinite desire   the collective shadow

a pendant around each throat
or a machine's toothed belt   replacing stillness with grasping

which feels like isolation
mesh and emptiness   meanwhile the real problem

is   to have a life these days is to walk around
with one's rage coagulating   around a deep wound

to exist inside   an increasingly attenuated
publicized self

in the office buildings' columned shadows
workers transfigure into shoppers

as something feudal hovers
darkly unhappy   alive

on the highways I spend
my body to the dregs but still   my body fails to comply

this lightning in my wrists   where damaged nerves crackle
this egg-shaped moon-ache in my low back

once I worked so much my lungs grew inflamed
and I nearly succeeded in disappearing

this was when I knew it   whatever *it* is   was near
like the realm's coins buried in a drawer

I would like to feel at home in the world
though I cannot

this knife of a translation
the animal flailing/failing   inside of me   a problem

Fear Song

This institution   heavy with
orderly sentences

moves as   a whole crowd or conference
of flailing people

where understanding the rules
is a privilege   a secrecy

and obeying the rules
a circle of red light   implanted under the skin

emitting cues and alarms
across the body's wet dirt

its layers of fat
which are dark rooms of survival

how can I navigate   or at least that's what
I understood   what they said   was necessary

as something feral and competitive   moves across the crowd
the space collapses   tightens

with the decaying feeling
of surveillance and debt

packaged back to us
as marbled enlightenment   you know   *enlightenment*

which has already taken   so much from me
how much more will I allow it to take?

I think   gazing out the windows beyond
the lecture hall's podium

where a snowy mist descends
like an unmooring   a forgetting

outside this room   this tower of experts   there is
a winter field light   this is a test

Debt

After unpacking my new knives
and curtains   my purchased packages
I go to my new rented window   hungry   I go
to my dark window still dissatisfied
still scared   and suddenly
the feeling that something is out there
descends   like a black synth sound
who is outside   circling my house?
once I followed   for hours around a city
a truck with a sign that read *the way out*
I had been walking around
looking at other people's properties
feeling like   there was a secret language I was
supposed to learn   a long time ago
but never did and now it is too late
a thick animal musk fills the kitchen
I want to forget what it was I forgot
some deep miscalculation   some oversight
I want this poem to go away

Buy It for Life

By which I mean   you can't
under the laws of entropy   to which

real life mechanical objects are subject
just like   everything else

abandoned rowboats decompose
in blue seagrass

a damp circle of gray   electric lamps
a mouthful of eggs and I

admit to fatigue   or failure   or both
a cellular programming

shudders   a soft
cavity fills with cells

predetermined was it there all along
a throb along the timeline   are you good

at evading illness   will you have for yourself
a long life   preparing and hooded   days when

I am arrogant and therefore okay
days when I've gone   so far into

Time Sickness

When my mother turns her back but still
she needs help with her hospital gown so I glimpse
the hard black lumps   the purple lines
when the surgeon steps back to admire
not my mother   but his sculpting of her
when there is no room here
to doubt the decision
though   weeping   I doubted it
this trade for longevity
another 30 to 40 years of her life
which is still not enough
when my mother can never die because then
I will die too
when a new era begins
and behind us we hear   a darkness at the door
when blackberries perfume
the hot August forest
when only one thing matters   though I cannot
tell you what that is
when   flinging myself from task to task
an urgency accumulates
inside my body as inflammation
and exhaustion feels like
the only safe place   when the linear brain
experiences time as guilt
when each year more debris
blows into the basement
as the earth takes it all back   and sickness
is the only word we have for this process
thus we explain time
by way of sickness   and fear
when one day   I will have to live
without her   this is true
I am always grasping

and never really learning
in the maze of illuminated bridges
one long grope in the wet streets
when it is incredible
how many potential accidents
do and do not occur daily
how gentleness arrives
when least expected
and how people   try to find one another
inside crowds like heavy stars
when I so love who I love
bewildered by stillness these repeated half-deaths
when will I find
a different occupation   what
will I do one day   when my hands are so empty

Bloodline

Sequins shedding from a dress   my voice
disappears across the house

the creek in the ditch   widens
into a moat   bone-marrow green

and two women screaming
at each other outside my room

accumulates as a restlessness
inside my hands   overstimulating as static

downstairs a man cries   while the others bang around
in their infinite weathers

as a child I would find
the smallest place in the house   or would stiffen and force

the painful scene to blur   into shadow
something not yet   decided into being

in which   some feelings are mine and some
are everything already dead

agitated I am   served tea
am billowed   to soothe

I will conquer   this island I think   retreating into myself
with a wintering   my bluff

but outside the green
waters   rock sickly bright and rock

Sleepwalker

A heavy sleep beneath old furs   a familiar weight
it is very livable

I give myself up and wear it gladly
the shadowed thought parts   to reveal

a terrifying stillness   like opening
a glowing silence   inside a fridge at night

or to find inside a mirror   some wind
I walk the empty business sector at night

trailing my hand along chain-link
the concrete buildings emit a dull yellow fog

I cannot hold abundance
though I am good at attending to

the daily required appearances
to prove   I am still a normal woman

which is like a dark compliment
like a nationalism

a station   dim   in a country somewhere
which I do remember though I was barely there

sucking on the quiet of a wildness   so desperate I was
straining at my own fatigue

these days feelings are smaller
I throw them on with some relief at their smallness

the neon lilac freedom and the raging's
porous thresholds

are too much   it is easier
to be nowhere   and I recognize these ruins

Failed Search Party

To replace absence with noise
is one kind of failure

like forcing one's flushed cheek upon another's
the irresistible swaying breath

afterward we stomp around
the cabin attending to things

a skinny branch grows
an animal's drooping haunches

this craving to be moved by a story
if only narrative moved through the world

with us and our solitude
but does anything accumulate

without suspicion   and is what we perceive
only what we are at present feeling?

let me just say I do have
my hesitations   do regret

the fraying temperatures like
falling columns of wolves

I have such
a terrible hunger

returning outside often
to blow into my palms

to scan the dark erratically
with my violent flashlight

Rest Cure

I.

If longing is the color then I want
to see what lies on the other side of hunger

if surveillance is the color then vigilance
is the shape   and if the shape

is childhood's
winter night in the body

and surveillance is   the American landscape's
shadow in the house

eventually I discover   I have no shape
and I have a shape   and it is a flame

II.

Women shutting themselves
in bedrooms for days   the old family stories go

she was so tired she stayed home from the party
we thought it was just a bad cold

she wasn't really sick she was just anxious
she just willed herself   into getting sick

the narratives like   blades wrapped in cloth
labor's bruises in a box   passed under the table

to be frightened of rest like this
to be frightened of acquiescing

or of what happens
in breast tissue over time

how often the lymphs in my throat swell
how my brother has had inflammation cut

many times from his body
the scar on his throat   on his chest

I had a childhood ritual of watching
the women in my family undress

revealing their missing body parts   a loose bra cup
puffed skin sewn into borders

I look in the mirror and have a morbid thought
picture my breasts

someday sliced cleanly off
folded and burned like heavy wings

mythologies and their jeweled messages
hang loud in the air   like beaded curtains

I part their weight   on the other side
the room is dim and heavy with smoke

III.

I wake from a nap to silence
the shadow-darkened house   a cup of rainwater

my mother in her bathrobe
leaning limp over a doughnut on the couch

a quiet and lackluster eating   so not like her
the angle of sweat beneath her voice

I want a soothing hand to reach in
from the exterior and hold me down

IV.

So now   how does
my exhaustion

which is   the exhaustion of daily allegiance to
capitalism   harm others?   how does

my urgency   perpetuate my own and others'
exploitation?   and you know

what I am actually tired of? I am tired
of making men feel good about themselves

like   how much energy do I actually expend
demonstrating to men that I am listening?

the answer is   a lot
after work today I will find

some moss   neon green
to look into for awhile

and I will text my mother
who worked through her breast cancer and who

will never be able to retire
mama get some rest tonight   it's okay mama   it's okay

soft dark the orange   scent of cedar in winter
I wear my anger like

a buttery and creased   inherited leather
certainly it is impossible   to keep silent forever

Nothing Is As Dark As an Island

Like a loose horse
on a northern beach   I am strange and stunned

by my capacity for shapeshifting
and by grief's transmutations

which are just   the self's vowels
released into oceanic darkness

where nothing is calculable
and the night's weight   a dark sapphire animal

drinks from the human world
the sound of wind   or a wingbeat

the Pacific's dark rise
moves with a tender anarchism   shapeless at the bite of us

courage!   the little scrying tool says   and I am trying
mostly   but for   my white-knuckled grip

at the edge   of the dissolution of self
which is a soundless chasm opening

this fatelessness which demands
a release of power nothing

not loyalty to family systems
nor to men   nor to some dying   economic law's

dictations for what
I am and what constitutes a life can survive

I've heard that   buried in every timeline
are portals into others

which one day you might simply
step through   only realizing much later

that you did step through
and were thus transformed

Recurring Dream

Some message of future ease   vaguely familiar strangers
knock on my door   offering me fruit   gleaned

from my own trees but baked
into tarts   of strange and unknowable shapes

Formlessness

The viewer looks for herself in other women's bodies
a quiet fragmentation or destabilization

the viewer casually scrolls and wants
crystallizes boredom   the viewer she belongs

to a specific nation
distraction economics rustle   a busy landscaping

inside of which it is hard to recognize
the mysterious presence

hovering behind us   just there   and there
was grief all along

the viewer's feminine gaze   constructs a thin tent
of possible selves   another location's

stars looking so intentional
so cubed in heightened colors   where

does she get her confidence
this luminosity enticing as a white egg   as marble

Images

Today I put objects down pick others up   eat some food
accomplish a couple of things   then pause

unmanned at the sink   feel whatever about
my face as something dull

like *oh here it is again*   walking around and just there
wanting to be congratulated

and here is a pretty but boring photograph:
lemons   an Italian terrace   a blue and white porcelain bowl

like viewing a neon sunset through an iron lattice
deep listless   burnout under the patriarchy

the capacity for pleasure   a green color
draining from my body

when we are told each moment of empire
should have a glittering purpose in this life

can I sit with the way being eventless feels
when I am wild inside this box

Her Body

Just as an abstract line feels linguistic
the impulse to imagine her belly

rolled as she sits   is she imaginary or not   or small
how small   how quickly to sum

these kinds of things up   what does she
consume daily   rich eggs   citrus details

the shoulder's flexing shell   extended underside
of her wrist a shallow green bowl

almost certainly erotic the obsession
with her essence's colors

peach and blue
creamy tangerine   pale olive

meanwhile I try to fit my thighs   red and scarred
inside this sharp bright grid

I go everywhere with this difficult
man-made cylinder   a weapon   having been weaponized

I guess I am trying to be an attractive person
I guess that's the weird goal!

just as seeds require adaptive mechanisms
wind   water   other animals

I find these glass particles
in my yard and in my body   they multiply

as I touch each person in anxiety or
I don't know   in self-dispersal   yieldedness

Elemental Nouns

How to arrange myself in a pleasing
yet adequately compelling way

how does interiority fare
when I walk through the world   touching things

green stalks   real running water
scent of plain noodles

bright squares to translate void   I need this tethering
in order to not float   right off the surface

in the concrete night   a moon silence shining
like a distant perfume bottle

as a woman drinks sweet milk from a can
scratches a bug bite on her ankle

elsewhere a woman sweeps
an illuminated doorway   cuts wood and metal   I like

to see what kind of day someone is having
there are so many different ways to have a day

just this once I let my shirt open
by the dark stream so actually delicious I

nearly forget my face   then
the decision to take a photo against this blue   is this

interesting enough
is this   is this

Apologies Regarding Spatial Reasoning

A man imparts knowledge
onto/unto me   when I return to a common expectation

in the city's constructed air   where I owe
the public beautiful things   am always in debt

so I offer my questions   my interest
which require large energy reserves   shimmering   nuanced

sometimes they   the men   are not really doing
anything wrong

they are simply everywhere and large
enjoying things with ease and I can't help but notice

when a man cuts in front of me   it's like
yes you are a large man aren't you

before I step aside into some bushes
to create room   apologies

are always on the tip of my tongue   they just love
to jump out!   and I am tired

of feeling sorry for my presence
there are real things I love   like I love when

lamps switch on at night   I love
the lamps' green darkness   and I love

the windows like tide pools   which
let the darkness in

Disrupted

That is not a window
but a circle cut in concrete   the desire to consume

smoldering like an expensive holiday
what I have been for a long time becomes real

as I walk through glass and metal landscapes
the taste of badness in my throat   bags filled with receipts

to avoid the building's shadows which are so like faces
that is not a spell but some money

stuffed inside a sad mouth   and that is not rest
but a white noise machine muscling us

into sleep   in the cradle of almost middle-class
and these clothes I bought are not new costumes

but very old longings not wildness
but a dark hole in the city filled with lights

when suddenly a plateau of fire sharpens the darkness
burns through the fabric like

what I knew would come back and come back
shapeless animal of collective grief to which I was so cruel

It's Hard to Tell Who One's Enemies Are

I bite off a hard square of glowing residue
expect the world to respond accordingly

the shape within the shape
though it's not the world's fault

it's not anyone's   it's an imprecise and placeless rage
like banging one's head against

the tiny workings of the day as viewed
through this painful filter

where even the air itself
carries something suspicious

and I want everything to cohere
though things don't

another day   rushed and rusted
another institution   exercises its power

my touch swims
in the pulpy blindness of it

I've Struggled with a Language

Water allies   rain-carved   a sieve
of tasteless seeds   and a community obeys

the logic of its landscape
a molding sign reads   *no parking / I will shoot any invalids!*

one winter my brother walks so much he carves
a ring of mud around the house like a spell

at sunset a woman calls for her dog   into the blank sealight
how or what is a place refusing to yield to you?

after my marriage ends I feel
everything and nothing

I cry into my scarf
while a drunk couple throws glass bottles

at each other in their driveway and seagulls
smash purple shells on the docks

the ferries lit up like floating cakes
and city lights across the water   illuminate my fear

of being always on the periphery   on the outside of
life as I feel myself to be   and on the inside of   an old grief

this too is institutional   historical
the perpetual urge to flee

to prevent an inactivity so immobile it ritualizes
to compliance   I run every night

around the lampless park
stubborn   frightened   imagining each

evergreen a crouched man   this fear so familiar it has
blood-quickened into biological process

locked gleam of winter fatigue   chain-link
around an empty lot

bone-white clams emptied and heaped   I cannot
keep still   longing for leap after leap

like a wild imaginary   cloud-blue
don't you want that too?

it's a very northern fear   the fear of one day just
disappearing

into the damp woods'
singular mossy darkness   unspecified

when all your life you are told
of an inevitable family order   a limited filament

and the insidious whiteness of settlement
this is my lineage which I refuse to worship

I kneel but I refuse to drink   I kneel
unworshipfully

even if it was little more than nothing
I made of this year what I could

Everything I Purchased Today

What is so boring is that everything
washes itself in an ordinary light   business

as usual conducts itself through us
as my finger hovers   over *buy now* and why not

why not stand here hands on my hips surveying
my lands like a man!

the city pumps out   sentimental visuals
and I admit I am moved I kiss everything inside

I lift my face to something
big and oiled and sun-filled

little plastics fly in the moneyed wind   in fact
everything I touch is plastic   discarded

inside of which my grasping   bankrupt feeling
is a cultural artifact   the emotional runoff

of this unsustainable century   artificial light
what can we do if all we are is produced?

to buoy the aura as it cracks at the rim
it is pure frenzy   it is a drowning

hooked on something sweet
hands deep in my square of front yard

on occasion a dark bone feeling
interrupts and I wonder what   I am adding to or up

The Many Panics of This Century

Deep inside some problem of self-perception
a human face believes very much in its own importance
charges its electronics often
when a face finally alights upon
the desired object it buys all of it
to have too much of many good things
to know that everything can be undone
this is how a small life can be as prepared as possible
hoarded goods   a kettle of rusted water
to secure against winter's lightlessness
or what if again long travel approaches
on highways wedged/pressed
between hot machines   the brown dust on fire
to which a human face can respond like
a scared domestic thing or like
a crazier animal
what if it cannot be returned
what if the direction can't be taken back

Nursery Rhyme

The bar's hot air   strung through with eyes
forces the mind to both desensitize

and sharpen   a knife against whetstone
as the manuscript of the self loosens

rearranging myself like laundry I am traveling across
this space when a man

reaches out and flicks my nipple
then he and his friends laugh

and suddenly I am constructed
a summary of parts to be evaluated: tits ass thighs waist

when my body transformed
from childhood's privacy into observation

open to comments
an acceptable topic of family conversation even!

because I could not keep it contained
in the right shape

I was no longer ashamed but became
shame   learned the impossibility of privacy

clothed in other people's approval what I fear most now
is my own mind   is sitting with myself

over the years other voices grew louder until my own
interiority was extinguished

finally recognizing this lack
feels like a kind of freedom

and I find that I am angry
and the anger song   it goes like this

Festival Object

A woman without breasts walks the desert
her chest wrapped in shining scars like purple cords

her flower tattoos burst outward
and men offer admirations

they like her tattoos   you know
because she has suffered   but is still a compelling

pretty slip of physicality   owed to anyone/everyone
then picked clean like a human ocean

like mythologies what we revere
tells so much about ourselves

a certain smooth face for example
can command a crowd

a magic cabinet collects
this fetishized system of values

the man I am sleeping with
tells me this story   *isn't she a badass*

she's a cancer survivor and makes it sexy
he says   expecting a certain reaction

though my reaction is
for the image-self to disappear

an interior hum   *I don't want*
I don't want to be looked at   I don't want to be looked at
    anymore anymore

Self-Portrait from Inside a Tent, Against Wind

These perhaps   tiny wildnesses arrange themselves
beyond the structure

here a blurred wooded edge
here an approximate lake

nothing can prepare you for the self
reads a sticker on a woman's laptop

and it's true I am   a leap like a forest light
cloth pouring into wind

like a thick liquid   purpled   dimmed
a shook hollow space   a creamy bell

here what glows vertical
here the line or ladder wavers or climbs   into soft field

a figure with a small   curve of face I barely
recognize   and another thing at the colorless edge   and another

Performances

Honestly if I could choose I would be
the largest and most terrifying bird   not to be measured
by thin line after thin line
this is to protect myself from shattering
into sheer tenderness and wonder
I've never had consistent feelings about anything
except sincerity   which I would like to fight for
a friend says if she hears one more reference
to a woman opening   she will vomit
and I agree because I would love
to close more things
like doors to private spaces and like
my dumb face   which insists on staying open
each evening I need time to sort and rearrange
to move my big bags into a new room
while I shiver through the world
the pink sky of high desert plains calms me
entrusted with cradling
a pink cloud   which leaks from my arms
strangers make me weep   I cannot explain
and I am going to the field
though it's all   already over

Rent Is Due

Lately reminders of how little I own
what the world is actually   a big complicated edge

a contemporary object in the sky
the rooms where I have asked to live

suddenly out and about
on a Friday   I participate

through constant monetary exchanges   a mood
of ownership   errands

that will not affect my life really
what costs zero dollars   short-lived sightings

of butterflies   bird calls
the tiniest energetic vessels

my face also costs nothing
though this statement is arguable and confusing

at dusk occasional free information sinks
into the simple mountains

I am fine like this
surprised to be drying my hair in the short sun

Paprikás Csirke

Soft underside of an animal
a shadowed glow   this golden-orange broth

swirled almost confectionary   with sour cream
green peppers coaxed into translucence

paprika and oil   russet-colored as tiny liquid sunsets
pooling around the dark salty meat

which has   since I was little
made my mouth water   and which my ancestors brought here

wrung-out as dishrags
alongside their bloodied histories   their medieval fatigue

and their unexamined determination to find safety
in adhering to the rules of whiteness/violence

these prismed fragments sink   like wreckage
in the ocean-thick sleep of myself

so deeply that sometimes I freeze
in the middle of a task   paralyzed with indecision and terror

or skip meals for days and days
or feel my mind suddenly crumple   fragment into grief

or my chest fill   with bladed wings
little panicked bird   what would you like to release?

but I am trying to be tender and understand
where the violent systems live inside my body

I fold boiled cabbage leaves
into pale green packages   like spring foliage

or like steaming propaganda pamphlets left in rain
they fall open   so soft

with peppery meat and tomato
so bright red they are almost   an ancestral song   somatic

inheritance is a waning oil   perhaps only
spent energy's fumes

here I am eating until full   and taking up space
as my grandmothers before me could not

My Hunger Is Complicated

It matters   the number of women in the room
the technicians the doctors all women   who are discussing
someone's daughter   who's in Paris
and you know what   good for her
I like it when women are doing well
though I am an uncertain mirror
and I would like to forgive this sickness of my mothers
and I appreciate uneventfulness
when I lay down and the room
rustles around me but without me
and god I love it   when women bring other women things
one evening in Paris I watched a woman
bring her friend a glass of red wine in bed   then tuck her in
as I leave the hospital into broad blue sun   women
are outside happily   eating cold pasta and sandwiches
a new architecture with a nationless glow
and along the shore women
in their heavy bodies   in bathing suits   in sparkling water
so much fucking delight
oh it kills me a little   so much

Lake with Undetermined Outlets

At the party I knife through the rooms
looking for someone to sleep with

in one room   a brimming nectar
a dark-haired stranger with his back to me

in another the cool   mountainous scent of rain
sends a shock of pleasure so

unsettling I waver
inside my shape   my form flickering

like an unsteady image   so close to that extra
hidden dimension   that recklessness again

converted then into longing
like a tangerine rope curling out into nothingness

removes me from reality and afraid of loss I touch nothing
trying to remember what I wanted to remember

a beloved's words in the dark   in a hotel by the lake
my friend's breasts   her long geometric glow

each late spring's twilight the exact
dark green of cold grass   so erotic I find it

honestly painful   this life   and its capacity for surprise
and pleasure   is a bruise

each room is a house   and each house a bottomless lake
I search for contemporary acts of pleasure

in the sustained ugliness of the city that I could find
wildness even in the air

when all day I am hungry   remembering the way the lake shook
and the shape becomes a hum

Your Desire for a Consistent Reality Is Constantly Thwarted

A pinkish-orange light
approaches from the sea

the light goes out as it flies over the community
then the disorienting orange dusk

an undercurrent shivers   a woman embroiders
her own disruption   transfigures into

a manic light   the most direct form of herself
the new structurelessness

ranges mammalian   for sure   every city
has always hosted this low hum

but now no longer theory   we are required
to accept what we did not think we could

no one believed it   people hired to strategize said that
to reject this system would only require another bad system

but a second moon   necessitates its own rules
the exit only illuminated when cut from the lack of an exit

meanwhile invisible travelers   at the periphery
carry their little lamps   like ladders across a dark gap

Bloodline

A woman in Budapest is getting along just fine
rides the metro   buys tea and peppers

her little cloth bag illuminated   the pink glow
of rose doughnuts   poppyseed   sour cherry cake

other women wrapped in blankets wait for the bus
in deep summer   the rain plantlike

every evening the city unfolds like a crumb-filled napkin
airing its mild daily complaints

there is a shape
though not the one we think

a half-light moving
through ourselves the witnesses   we are not arcs

The Wild Under the Wilderness

Touching the dune grasses and their tall glow
an easy way to locate oneself

I have a pile of something here   elemental nouns
which disperse   like seasonal insects

quinces poach in pink cinnamon syrup
plant cuttings on the windowsill embroider

water with soft roots   and suddenly I am more
committed to everything than I realized

isn't this just
so consistently my weakness   that I want to stay

stay here I mean   on earth
accumulating these little houses

and I tie this old   childhood love around my waist
while I wade out farther and I wade out farther

Returning Home in Late Spring

To believe the world can be unbuilt
you have to trust yourself

I write on the back of my hand   after a long illness
I take an evening boat into the city

my face almost frightening in its plainness
opened by fever into pure   vulnerability

in mists and emerald-dark spruces
people hurry home carrying meat

a familiar landscape sloughs off fragments
of emotional information   I can see the unstable shards

shimmer in orange-wet air   tempted as I am
to gather them I am   unlearning

thus the world moves through me like money   the world
moves through me like something that does not belong to me

on the dock I say hello to someone I secretly
loved in high school and feel fine

feel light even   like a confident party guest
ambivalence's ornateness   so satisfying

a brushed black spring night
the moon on the water's   cold green surface

I am tired of trying to be an easy person
to be around   like

what if I tried to be a difficult
person to be around?   illegible   unpredictable

as fire separated from sun   and for a little rage
to succeed occasionally   is that too much to ask

effortless in warm weather   loosened as silk
as failures will do to the self

I row home with my strong back
a handful of coastal strawberries

with the red scent of burning pine in my hair
and with my anger   my power

Notes

This book would not have been possible without the mentorship, love, and wisdom of Ruth Ellen Kocher—thank you for truly seeing and nurturing my work and my voice, Ruth.

Thank you to other faculty at the University of Colorado Boulder who generously read early versions of this manuscript: Noah Eli Gordon, Julie Carr, Elisabeth Sheffield, and Kelly Hurley. And thank you to Sandra Yannone at The Evergreen State College for giving me the energy and courage to complete the final push to find this book a home in the world.

I am equally grateful to my beloved creative community who read and provide feedback for my work, and who keep me writing: Katie Woods, Loie Rawding, Rushi Vyas, Aaron Klass, Thomas Ross, and others.

Thank you to my cousin Hannah Brancato for inspiring and energizing me since we were children, for collaborating on our creative projects and workshops, and for making this book's cover art.

Thank you to the scholars, activists, and artists who taught me as I wrote, especially Resmaa Menakem and Carlin Quinn, whose somatic abolitionism workshop with Education for Racial Equity deeply transformed me and influenced this book. Many of the lines and ideas in "Fear Song" were inspired by their teachings.

Thank you to my family and their tireless interest in and encouragement of my work: Ian and Steph, Hunter, Duncan and Sharron, and Jane and Mike.

Acknowledgements

Grateful acknowledgement to the following journals where many of these poems first appeared, often in different forms, under different titles:

Bennington Review, "I Am a Bad System"

Black Warrior Review, "Village"

Colorado Review, "Rent Is Due"

Columbia Poetry Review, "Formlessness," "Arrival"

Crazyhorse, "Interior vs. Exterior," "Lineage of Power"

The Feminist Wire, "Elemental Nouns," "A Room"

Heavy Feather Review, "Disrupted"

Hobart, "The Many Panics of This Century"

Ilk, "Failed Search Party"

Matter Monthly, "The Tarp"

Mississippi Review, "A Childhood"

Poetry Northwest, "Returning in Late Summer to the Uncanny"

Prelude, "The Knife"

Quarterly West, "Apologies Regarding Problems with Spatial Reasoning"

Smoking Glue Gun, "Milk"

Typo, "Performances"

Yalobusha Review, "Your Desire for a Consistent Reality Is Constantly Thwarted"

"Failed Search Party," "The Water Effect," and "Bloodline (Sequins shedding across the house...)" also first appeared in the chapbook *Geography* (dancing girl press, 2015).

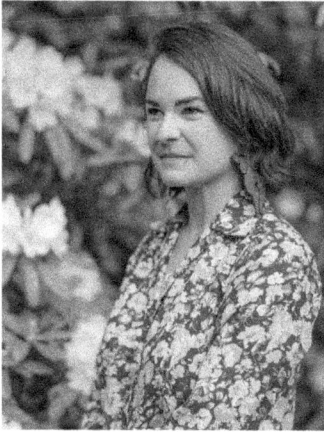

About the Author

Ansley is a writer and teacher from the Pacific Northwest. She holds an MFA in Poetry from the University of Colorado Boulder and is the author of the chapbook *Geography* (dancing girl press, 2015). Her work has appeared in *Poetry Northwest*, *Colorado Review*, *swamp pink*, *Bennington Review*, and elsewhere. She currently works as the Director of the Writing Center at The Evergreen State College and teaches poetry and mixed media workshops at local community arts organizations, including Hugo House in Seattle. She lives in Olympia, Washington with her dog.

www.ingramcontent.com/pod-product-compliance
Lightning Source LLC
Chambersburg PA
CBHW022102020426
42335CB00012B/794